Hemp Oil and CBD

The Absolute Beginner's Guide to CBD and
Hemp Oil for Better Health, Faster Healing
and More Happiness

TIMOTHY GREENE

DEDICATION

To my friend Chris

CONTENTS

INTRODUCTION

I want to thank you for choosing this book, 'Hemp Oil and CBD - The Absolute Beginner's Guide to CBD and Hemp Oil or Better Health, Faster Healing and More Happiness.'

Cannabis is one of the most versatile plants in nature and yet considered illegal in several parts of the world. This is mainly owing to the mood altering effects that it can have on a person's mind. However, cannabis does not always have psychoactive effects on the brain and, instead, produces some of the most powerful medicinal oils and by-products in the world such as hemp oil and CBD.

Right from enhancing skin quality to curing cancer, hemp oil and CBD provide a plethora of health benefits, where just a little goes a long way in enhancing well-being. But hemp oil and CBD are not easily available thereby making it difficult for people to exploit their benefits.

In this book, we will delve into the details of hemp oil and CBD to understand exactly how you can use them to enhance your health.

Let us begin.

CHAPTER 1: HEMP OIL AND CBD EXPLAINED

First and foremost, I thank you for choosing this book and hope you have a good time reading it. In this first chapter, we will look at the meaning of hemp oil and CBD, and understand how they work on the body.

What is hemp oil?

Hemp oil is a medicinal oil that is extracted from hemp plants. Although all plants in the cannabis family can produce oils, hemp is predominantly used to extract oil used for medicinal purposes. Hemp plants have lesser THC as compared to other plants in the same genus. THC is the compound that has psychoactive effects on the mind. It is, therefore, safe for use and is extracted to produce an oil that has countless medicinal properties.

How is it sourced?

Hemp oil is mostly extracted from the seeds of the hemp plant. Although the entire plant can be used to extract oil, the best quality comes from seeds. The seeds are cold pressed to extract oil. It is light green in color and has a nutty flavor to it. It then undergoes a simple refining process that renders the oil colorless. The oil is not processed further and manufactured as it is, to preserve concentrated levels of CBD. Unrefined hemp oil does not have good shelf life and must be used within days of being pressed. However, hemp plant cannot be grown legally in many parts of the world thereby making it a rare herb. Several countries put it in the same category as other cannabis plants thereby causing its price to remain on the higher side.

How does it work on the body?

Hemp oil contains several chemicals that are good for the body. Right from helping with skin rejuvenation to curing cancer, hemp oil contains vital nutrients that penetrate deep into skin and benefit organs, cells etc. Hemp oil mostly finds its use in topical treatment and is regarded as an effective means to deal with aches and pains.

What are its benefits?

Hemp oil is used in several industries such as the beauty industry. It is added to creams and lotions as also soaps and toiletries. Hemp oil has been used since time immemorial to rejuvenate skin and deal with conditions such as acne and psoriasis. Hemp oil is also used in the making of gels and creams to combat aches and pains. The oil is quite powerful and penetrates deep into the skin to provide instant relief. Hemp oil is also used as a dietary supplement, as it contains high levels of fatty acids that are great for maintaining heart health.

What is the nutritional value of hemp?

Hemp oil contains 75-80% polyunsaturated fat and only about 8 to 10% unwanted saturated fat. This makes it one of the healthiest oils in the world capable of enhancing overall health. Unsaturated fatty acids contained in the oil are not naturally produced by our bodies thereby making them extremely useful. Although certain foods that we eat contain these essential fatty acids, we mostly end up not getting the right amount. Just with a little addition of hemp oil to our meals, we can successfully make up for the deficit, and ensure we get the right dose of unsaturated acids.

Is it safe for use?

Yes. Hemp oil can be safely used both internally and externally. The chemicals contained within the oil are skin friendly and will not lead to any form of adverse reaction. However, it will be advisable to do a patch test if you have sensitive skin. You will also have to consult a physician if you consume any medications. If you have any allergies then it is best to first check with your doctor before using hemp oil for cooking purposes.

What is CBD?

CBD stands for cannabidiol. This is a chemical that is predominantly present in cannabis plants. CBD, unlike THC or tetrahydrocannabinol, does not have any psychoactive effects on the brain. This, therefore, makes it safe for use and is used in the preparation of medicines, creams, lotions etc. CBD was overlooked by the medical community for a long time as it was often confused with THC. But over the course of several years, CBD's true medicinal properties were discovered thereby pushing it towards mainstream usage.

How is it sourced?

CBD can be extracted from cannabis plants including hemp and marijuana. Most people grow marijuana plants in order to harvest the leaves and decarboxylate them to enhance the CBD contained within it. CBD is manufactured on a large scale and used in many factories such as cosmetic companies.

How does it work?

CBD is one of 80 chemicals that are present inside cannabis leaves and seeds. CBD is a chemical that does not have psychoactive effects on the brain but benefits the body in many different ways. These cannabinoids attach to cannabinoid receptors in the body, most of which are found in the nervous system. They are also found in skin, digestive system and reproductive systems. These receptors can be sensitive and absorb CBD quickly. The cell receptors absorb cannabinoid and form a complex internal network known as endocannabinoid system. These are regarded as one of the body's greatest neurotransmitter systems. Once absorbed, CBD almost immediately begins work on the body.

What are its benefits?

CBD is an extremely effective chemical that affects the body in many different ways. It is regarded as one of the best natural supplements to consume as it enhances overall bodily function. Cannabinoids are known for their anti-inflammatory properties. CBD also has antioxidant properties that make it ideal for the upkeep of cell health. CBD is an anxiolytic and antidepressant and used in the treatment of depression and anxiety. CBD has analgesic properties and finds its use in the treatment of infections. The chemical also has anti-tumoral and antipsychotic effects on the body thereby making it quite versatile.

Is it safe for use?

Yes. CBD supplements are safe for use. They can be administered to a variety of people including elders, children and adults. However, it would be advisable to consult a physician first, to make sure the diet is safe to adopt.

CHAPTER 2: HEMP OIL BENEFITS

Hemp oil is rich in several vital nutrients that are capable of curing many illnesses. Here are some of the health benefits provided by hemp oil.

Hormonal balance

It is extremely important to maintain hormonal balance in the body, especially for women hitting menopause. Several factors including stress and poor diet increase chances of a hormonal imbalance that can lead to conditions such as PCOS, anxiety, depression etc. However, with the use of hemp oil, it is possible to restore hormonal balance and make it easier for women to maintain good health. Hemp seeds contain gamma-linoleic acid that gets converted to a protective hormone called prostaglandin, which regulates hormonal balance and supports women's bodies during menopause.

Skin health

One of the biggest health benefits provided by hemp oil is skin rejuvenation. Hemp oil contains omega 3 and 6 fatty acids that are comparable to skin lipids. This makes them excellent natural moisturizers that penetrate deep into the skin. Hemp oil is beneficial for dry skin, nails and hair. It is also a great choice for treating wrinkles, as it increases elasticity and makes skin smoother. Hemp oil is especially useful in winters when skin tends to dry out. Hemp oil is generally added to moisturizers, beauty creams, hair oils, gels, masks etc. A little hemp oil can be massaged into the skin on a regular basis in order to smooth it out and get rid of wrinkles.

Fatty acids

One of the biggest complaints that vegetarians and vegans have is the lack of food options that provide a good dose of omega 3 and 6 fatty acids. These are extremely important for well being and maintenance of heart health. In such a situation, hemp oil makes for the best choice, and a good alternative to fish oil. It contains omega 6 and 3 fatty acids in the ration 3:1, which is ideal for the maintenance of good health. Hemp oil has a pretty neutral taste thereby making it ideal to be drizzled over a variety of foods.

Heart health

The heart is one of the most important organs of the body, yet the most neglected. People do not realize the importance of maintaining good heart health and end up consuming foods that negatively impact it. One good way of ensuring good heart health is through the consumption of hemp oil and hemp oil supplements. It contains fatty acids that cut into built up cholesterol in the body and reduce chances of developing heart disease. You will have the chance to reverse some of the damage caused by the consumption of junk and processed foods and be in a good position to maintain a healthy heart. Your rate of metabolism will intensify thereby ensuring a breakdown of fat that does not have the chance to get deposited on artery walls.

Lean muscles

Hemp oil is rich in proteins thereby making it ideal for the development of lean muscles. Lean muscles are those that are not easily burnt away. Adding a little hemp oil to your meals before or after a workout can help in increasing chances of developing leaner muscles.

Diabetics

Diabetes is now turning out to be one of the biggest enemies of good health. Hemp oil can help in controlling the condition to a certain extent owing to its low sugar and carbohydrate content. It is also ideal for all who wish to keep diabetes at bay, especially those who have a predisposition towards it. Hemp oil can be drizzled over the foods, as it is quite versatile. It can be added to both vegetarian and non-vegetarian meals such as salads and soups.

Immunity

Hemp oil can be added to meals to enhance immunity. The oil helps in regulating intestinal flora thereby building a natural barrier against germs. This, therefore, enhances the body's disease-fighting capacity. Once you start consuming the oil, you will notice that you fall sick less often. You will also experience lesser joint aches and pains.

Nervous system

The nervous system is stimulated by fatty acids. These are essential for maintaining healthy cell membrane structure. These fatty acids prevent the demyelination, which refers to the destruction of the myelin sheath. This sheath protects the nerve cells. Just with the use of a little hemp oil, you will be able to relax your mind and body.

Varicose veins

Varicose veins is a condition wherein the veins present in legs begin to swell up and allow a backflow of blood. In such a case, it becomes important to thin the blood down so that it can easily flow upwards. Hemp oil, being rich in omega 3 fatty acids, can help in thinning blood. This helps in reducing clots and soothes varicose veins.

Precautions to observe

There are a few precautions to observe with hemp oil in order to ensure safe administration. They are as follows.

Anticoagulant

Hemp oil is an anticoagulant and therefore people who take blood thinners should avoid it. You can consult your doctor in case you wish to use hemp oil externally.

Prostate

Men who suffer from prostate issues should avoid using hemp oil. The oil is said to increase chances of developing a tumor.

High doses

It is important to avoid consuming hemp oil in high doses as it can lead to diarrhea, nausea and cramps. The ideal dose of hemp oil is 1 to 2 tablespoons per day.

Cooking

Avoid cooking with hemp oil, as heating it can lead to the conversion of unsaturated fat into saturated fat. It is ideal to drizzle the oil over salads and soups.

CHAPTER 3: CBD HEALTH BENEFITS

Like hemp oil, CBD also contains body-nourishing nutrients. Here is a look at some of the positive effects of CBD on your body.

Mood enhancement

CBD helps in enhancing mood. CBD has the tendency to relax your mind and improve blood circulation. It is especially useful for those who suffer from anxiety and depression. Just a little oil consumed on a daily basis can go a long way in reducing mental ailments. With regular use, you will feel less irritable and more productive.

Memory enhancement

CBD enhances memory. CBD supplements can be consumed on a daily basis, for a certain period of time, in order to improve memory and cognition. CBD contains certain chemicals that help in improving memory. It helps in relaxing the mind and can help those suffering from PTSD. It is beneficial for students, as they can use hemp oil to increase their memory power and remember better during exams. It is also ideal for older people who feel like their memory power is being affected by age.

Motor skills

Motor skills are those that are carried out when the brain, nervous system and muscles work in tandem. Motor skills can be enhanced through the use of CBD supplements. These skills tend to deteriorate over time and can lead to the development of certain ailments. The best thing to do in order to avoid such a situation is consuming CBD supplements so that it is easier to exercise control over your motor skills.

Immunity

CBD increases immunity. Immunity refers to the body's disease-fighting capacity, which can be enhanced through the consumption of CBD supplements. The liver happens to be the main organ that defends the body against germs. By consuming CBD, you have the chance to enhance liver function thereby increasing chances of warding off ailments. CBD also helps in keeping the gut healthy. With regular use, you can prevent both liver and gut ailments and remain in a good position to steer clear of common illnesses such as coughs and colds.

Reproduction

It is possible to increase your fertility through the use of CBD. CBD is said to be an aphrodisiac that improves libido. It is especially useful among those who suffer from re-productivity issues. Just a little oil, added to meals, on a regular basis can help people, suffering from fertility; reverse their condition to a certain extent. CBD oil is directly rubbed over the areas corresponding to reproductive organs in order to provide relief from fertility issues.

Pain

CBD is known to reduce pain threshold. Those who suffer from pain owing to conditions such as varicose veins and arthritis will experience a reduction through the consumption of CBD supplements. Oils rich in CBD can also be used to massage over the areas where a person experiences pain, as it helps in reducing the sensation. CBD consumed regularly also helps athletes strengthen their muscles and avoid the risk of sprain and muscle pull. A little CBD oil applied over the affected muscle can greatly help in reducing the pain and reversing the condition to a certain extent.

Appetite control

One of the best ways to control weight is by controlling appetite. CBD helps in controlling your appetite to a large extent. With regular consumption of CBD, you will not feel the urge to consume snacks in between meals. You will feel quite energetic throughout the day and have enough energy left to perform activities post work.

Sleep enhancement

Sleep happens to be a very important activity. When you sleep, your body repairs the various organs and ensures that they function optimally. Many people suffer from sleep deprivation owing to stress and wrong food habits. One great way of enhancing sleep is through the consumption of CBD supplements. CBD helps in not only increasing your sleeping capacity but also enhances your body's tendency to repair the various organs.

Healthier bones

Bone health is often neglected when it comes to maintaining a healthy body. It is important to pay attention to bone health, especially after a certain age. One good way of ensuring good bone health is through the consumption of CBD supplements. It helps in the absorption of calcium into the bloodstream thereby preventing calcium depletion from bones. Healthier bones translate to lesser injuries and the chance to lead a healthier, longer life.

Precautions to observe

It is advisable to avoid consumption of antacids 2 to 6 hours after consuming CBD supplements. It is best to avoid consuming dairy products as they can interfere with the drug. Those suffering from anxiety and depression must avoid consuming the supplement as it can agitate the condition. It will be best to avoid driving after consuming the drug.

CHAPTER 4: GROWING HEMP AND CANNABIS PLANTS, EXTRACTING CBD

As mentioned earlier, it is not legal to grow hemp and marijuana plants in several parts of the world. Please check with your local legislation before growing THC-rich plants. If it is legal in your country, you can grow your own hemp and marijuana plants at home to extract hemp oil and CBD.

Growing hemp plants

Hemp plants are fairly easy to grow. Here is how you can grow them.

Soil

Hemp can grow in a variety of soils. You can use black or red soil or a mixture of the two. But remember that the soil needs to be well drained and not hold water over the surface, as hemp plants do not do well in flooded environments. You can make a few small holes on the surface of the soil to ensure proper drainage.

Pots

You must use proper pots to grow hemp plants. It will be ideal to sow it in the ground but if you have a space crunch, then you can go for cement pots. They will be sturdy and not break as easily. They will also provide plants with proper support if in case you wish to grow them tall. Avoid using plastic pots, as they will not drain away water easily. Keep the pots covered during monsoons as otherwise, plants can wilt. Make about 3 1-inch deep holes in the soil and drop 2 seeds into each. Cover lightly with soil and water immediately. Plants will start to grow within 2 to 3 weeks.

Watering

It is best to water your hemp plants on alternate days. Wait for the topsoil to dry out before watering the plants. If there is too much water accumulated at the top then drain it away. Add nutrient-rich fertilizers once a week in order to enhance plant quality. Adding coco-coir to the top ensures retention of moisture and nutrients. A mixture of neem oil and water can be sprayed to the stem to avoid insect infestation.

Sun

The plants require a minimum of 4 hours of sun to grow properly. Place it in a spot where the whole plant can receive sunlight. If there is too much sun then move the pot to a shady area after 4 to 5 hours. Protect young plants from direct wind.

Harvesting

You must harvest your hemp as soon as the last pollen is shed by the plant. Once that is done, you have to wait for at least a month before harvesting the seeds. You have to harvest the leaves and seeds carefully so as not to damage the plant. Once the plant is harvested, you can leave it out to dry. You can use the process of retting to dry the stems. Leave them out in the sun for a few hours every day for a fortnight, turning them around every couple of days.

Growing Marijuana plants

Marijuana plant belongs to the same family as hemp plants. Marijuana contains more THC but can be harvested to extract CBD. These are easier to grow and can be grown indoors. Here's how you can do so.

Soil

Marijuana grows in a variety of soils including red and black soil. Marijuana plants tend to grow well in a mixture of black and red soil with a little neem powder mixed in. You can also grow them through a soil-less system known as hydroponics.

Pots

If you plan on growing them indoors, then it is best to pick small pots. These can be placed inside artificially created light zones. Plastic pots are better for indoor use. Make sure they are sturdy and well draining.

Lighting

It is best to create an artificial lighting environment for your marijuana plants, as they will grow better. Grow lights can be installed depending on the size of the garden. You can also invest in a tent to keep them confined to one corner of the room.

Watering

They can be watered on alternate days or as and when the topsoil dries out. Do not overwater the plants as that can lead to root rot. Sprinkling coco-coir on top ensures retention of water and nutrients.

Harvesting

Remember that only female plants produce the best crop. If you spot any male plants growing then it is best to remove them. Once the buds develop pink crystals, you can harvest the plants. Carefully pick out the leaves and buds and hang them to dry.

Decarboxylate

It is important to decarboxylate cannabis plants in order to strengthen the CBD content. Here is how you can do so.

- Preheat the oven to 240 degrees F.
- Cut the flowers, buds and leaves and spread them over a tray ensuring no area of the tray remains exposed.
- Do not cut them too small as they can burn. If you spot any small pieces then remove them.
- Place tray in the oven for 30 to 40 minutes or until the leaves turn crumbly.
- Remove from oven and wait for it to cool down completely.
- Place a few leaves and flowers between your palms to make a coarse powder.
- Add the powder to an airtight container.

The weed is now ready to use.

Extracting CBD oil

Here is how you can extract CBD oil.

Materials required:

- 1-ounce hemp or marijuana leaves
- 2 plastic buckets
- 1 wooden stick or spatula
- 2 cups Isopropyl alcohol
- 1 coffee filter
- 1 large container
- 1 rice cooker
- 1 ventilation fan
- 1 teaspoon water
- Oven mitts
- Stainless steel bowl
- Dehydrator
- 1 plastic bottle

Method:

- Ensure that everything is dry before starting the process.
- Use the alcohol to dampen the hemp or marijuana leaves.
- Now use a spatula to gently crush the leaves.
- Add in more solvent into the mixture such that it is covered. Gently mix everything in so that the CBD and THC content dissolve into it.
- Pour this out into bottles before adding in some more solvent and mix until the remaining CBD dissolves.
- Pour this mixture into the bucket and discard all the leaves.
- Pour this mixture through the coffee filter in order to separate any residual leaves.
- Next, you will require a rice cooker to burn the solvent (alcohol) away. But remember to do it in a well-ventilated room, as the fumes from the process can be quite toxic and inflammable.
- Fill the cooker with the mixture and plug it in. Turn the temperature to 140 C.

- If there is more space and you have some mixture left over then add that in as well.
- At this stage, add in about a teaspoon of water to the mixture as it prevents burning.
- At this stage, you are required to gently swirl the cooker so that all the solvent evaporates. But make sure you wear mitts so that you don't burn your hands.
- Once done, carefully pour the oil out into a steel bowl.
- Place this bowl on slow heat like a coffee warmer or dehydrator in order to heat up the oil.
- The oil will start bubbling and continue to do so for some time. Once the bubbles stop, the oil will be ready for use.

Tips to buy hemp oil

If you wish to buy hemp oil from the store then here are a few tips to bear in mind.

Quality

It will be important to buy good quality hemp oil to use for cooking. If you are buying it online, then you have to go through a trusted website. If you are buying from a store then make sure the oil is food grade and looks colorless. If possible, smell it to check whether any smell has been added into it.

Quantity

It is best to buy a small quantity of oil, as hemp oil does not come with shelf life. You restock on it as soon as it exhausts.

Price

Good quality hemp oil can be a little expensive. If you buy an inexpensive one then you will be compromising on the quality.

CHAPTER 5: SIMPLE HEMP OIL RECIPES AND COSMETICS

Here are a few simple recipes that you can try out using hemp oil.

Canna butter

Ingredients:

- 1 cup decarboxylated canna leaves
- 1 cup butter

Method:

- Line a baking tray with cling film.
- Add the butter and canna leaves to the blender and whizz until well combined.
- Add this to the baking tray and use a spoon or spatula to spread it around.
- Place in the fridge to harden completely.
- Remove from the cling film and use in place of regular butter.

Hemp oil pasta

Ingredients:

- 3 tablespoons hemp oil
- 1 tablespoon olive oil
- 8 ounces fettuccine, uncooked
- 4 cloves garlic, minced
- 2 cups chicken broth
- 1 cup milk, or more, as needed
- 1/4 cup Parmesan cheese, grated
- Kosher salt and pepper, as per taste
- 2 tablespoons fresh parsley leaves, coarsely chopped

Method:

- Bring the chicken stock to a boil and add in the pasta.
- Allow it to cook fully.
- Add the olive oil to a pan and allow it to heat up.
- Add in the garlic and sauté till brown.
- Add the salt and pepper and mix.
- Once the pasta is done, add it to the pan and toss.
- Add the pasta to a bowl and drizzle the hemp oil on top.
- Serve with a generous sprinkling of Parmesan cheese and parsley leaves on top.

Hemp oil salad

Ingredients:

- 1 small onion
- 2 small tomatoes
- 1 cucumber
- ¼ pineapple
- Mint leaves to sprinkle
- 2 tablespoons hemp oil

Method:

- Chop the onions and add to a bowl.
- Add in the tomatoes, cucumber and pineapple and mix till well combined.
- Sprinkle the mint leaves on top.
- Drizzle the hemp oil and serve.

Hemp oil vinaigrette

Ingredients:

- 3 tablespoons hemp oil
- 1 teaspoons lemon juice
- 1 tablespoon balsamic vinegar
- 1 tablespoon mustard
- 2 garlic cloves, minced
- Salt to taste
- Pepper to taste

Method:

- Add the hemp oil to a bowl along with the lemon juice and mix well.
- Add the balsamic vinegar and mustard and whisk until combined.
- Add the mustard and garlic and mix well.
- Add the salt and pepper and mix until well combined.
- Use as a dressing to pour over salads.

Hemp oil cream

Ingredients:

- 1 cup shea butter
- 5 tablespoons hemp oil
- 5 tablespoons lavender essential oil

Method:

- Add the shea butter to a double boiler and use a blender to whip it gently.
- Add in the hemp oil and mix well.
- Add the lavender essential oil and mix.
- Allow it to cool down before adding to an airtight container.

This cream can be applied to hands and feet.

Hemp oil lip butter

Ingredients:

- ½ cup shea butter
- ¼ cup beeswax
- 5 tablespoons hemp oil
- 2 drops vitamin e oil
- 2 tablespoons rose essential oil

Method:

- Add the shea butter and beeswax to a double boiler and melt gently.
- Add in the hemp oil along with the vitamin e oil and mix well.
- Add the rose oil and stir.
- Pour into a tub and or container and apply over lips.

Hemp oil for hair

Ingredients:

- 1 cup olive oil
- 1 cup hemp oil

Method:

- Mix the olive and hemp oil together and add to a bottle.
- Shake the bottle such that both oils mix well.
- Apply to roots and length of hair twice a week.
- Wash off after 1 hour.

CONCLUSION

I thank you once again for choosing this book and hope you had a good time reading it.

The main aim of this book was to educate you on the basics of hemp oil and CBD. As you can see, both are extremely useful and can be used to serve a variety of purposes.

Good luck!

– Timothy

46496604R00021

Made in the USA
Middletown, DE
01 August 2017